Easy

WEIGHT LOSS

JOAN MARIE

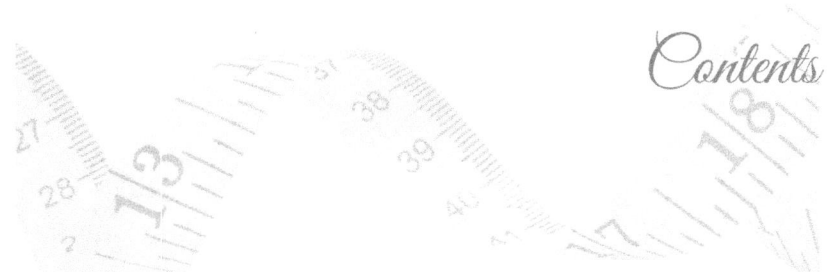

Contents

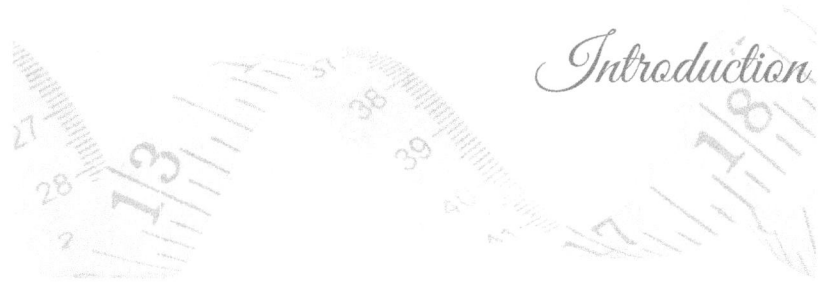

I was scared. I had just been diagnosed with breast cancer and my life flashed before me. Well, actually my life didn't flash before me. It was more like I was analyzing my life more now. I was forty eight years old and I thought to myself, *Is this it?* The lump in my breast had been there for quite some time, and I wondered how I could have been so out of touch with my own body to miss it.

I think when anyone hears the word "cancer" it is so terrifying that it almost doesn't register in the person's mind. I almost went numb inside. What was I going to do now? Oh my God— I was going to lose my hair! Then suddenly I realized, *who cares about hair, I may lose my life*!

I was middle aged and overweight. I had never realized how over-weight I was until I had to take a body scan, and I saw so much fat around my bone structure that I was shocked. I was never fat when I was young; back then I was 5'7" tall, I weighed between 135 and 145 pounds, and I wore a size 6 or 8—that is considered downright skinny for an African American female! But now I weighed over 200 pounds and I was wearing a size 14 or 16. I had let myself go, as some would like to say. But I really thought it was normal to gain weight in middle age, because when I looked at the women who surrounded me at that time, they were all overweight, and I was no different.

I just didn't understand that aging had nothing to do with weight gain; what I'm saying is this: if you eat healthy and exercise you will not become overweight, in most cases. We all hear that our metabolism slows down when we age, but that is not an excuse to become overweight.

I had done a lot of damage to my body with my diet. I ate steak, pork, chicken, white bread, ice cream and cakes on a regular basis. You see, I followed the SAAD, which stands for Standard African American Diet, for my entire life. And now I had breast cancer. And yes, it is my understanding and opinion that your diet has a lot to do with your health.

So I went through the operation to remove the tumor, and I went through chemo, and it was a very difficult time in my life. With the help of my very supportive husband and family, I got through it. But what many women don't know is that after their treatment, a type of fear can set in—the fear of a recurrence of cancer. Through many internet searches, I found that exercise and diet had a lot to do with keeping your body healthy and lowering the chances of a recurrence of cancer.

After treatment, I made a promise to myself that I would change my life. I mean really change! I started exercising and eating meat that was organic, and I changed the size of my portions. Then slowly I started eliminating chicken, beef, pork and turkey; I also started eating more vegetables. I started juicing and preparing smoothies that were full of good food with lots of nutrition. I also started to exercise by walking 30 minutes a day, either at lunch or in the evenings. And over about a 3-year period I went from size 14/16 to size 6/8. Oh yes, and I am healthier now and much happier.

Yes it took time, but I did it my way; it worked, and I kept it off! Not only that, I have been cancer-free for 10 years - yea! So now I want to help you do the same thing. I want you to know that you can lose the weight if you create your own personalized, tailor-made plan to do so. And know this—you can get your figure back no matter what age you are. I got mine back.

In this book I don't give you crazy diets or recipes or exercise routines. I give you an understanding of how to change your lifestyle. Changing your lifestyle is long-term, so you can take your time and enjoy the journey. Just remember one thing—it's really about getting healthy and preventing health-related issues. Focus on improving your health and you just might be pleasantly surprised when you start to reap one of the benefits of being healthy, which is weight loss.

May you continue to be blessed and find peace and love. And please enjoy your journey!

Genesis 1:29 New International Version (NIV)

29 Then God said, "I give you every seed-bearing plant on the face of the whole earth and every tree that has fruit with seed in it. They will be yours for food.

Exodus 23:25 New International Version (NIV)

25 Worship the Lord your God, and his blessing will be on your food and water. I will take away sickness from among you.

Chapter 1

BLACK WOMEN AND WEIGHT LOSS

I had to talk about this subject because black women don't look at being overweight as a serious health issue. Our culture welcomes overweight women, big butts and thick thighs. But if the big butts and thick thighs are overweight, this can cause major medical problems. Did you know that black women are more likely than white women to die from breast cancer?

Here are some facts I found in an article titled "More Black Women Are Dying from Breast Cancer than White Women—And the Disparity is Growing Every Year."

A new study found a huge racial gap in breast cancer mortality rates.

Published on March 20, 2014, by Casey Gueren.

"There is a significant racial disparity between black and white women in breast cancer-related deaths in the U.S., according to a new study published in the journal Cancer Epidemiology. And even more shocking is the fact that this gap became even wider in many cities from 1990 to 2009. These startling findings pose the question: Why are more black women dying from breast cancer than white women each year?"

The study also suggests that we aren't getting help early enough by getting our mammograms and doing our self-checkups, along with educating ourselves about the dangers of breast cancer.

JOAN MARIE

It is my opinion that if we get our weight under control, if we eat healthier meals and we start to incorporate exercise into our tailor-made weight loss plans, then we will, as black women, be leaders in getting rid of breast cancer.

Chapter 2

THE TRUTH ABOUT SOUL FOOD

So let's be honest, do you really think that soul food is good for you? I mean do you really think you can continue to eat fried chicken wings, hog mogs, chit lings, pig feet, greens cooked in animal fat and not get sick? The bible says my people die from lack of knowledge, so let me give you some knowledge to save your life.

Let's talk about the origins of soul food. It is my understanding that the term soul food became popular in the 1960s. We as African Americans thought nothing of it to eat pig feet and greens basically cooked in animal fat. It was something that was passed down to us, in other words we inherited this type of diet from our parents etc...

But we should know and understand that this diet is killing us, and we need to stop eating this deadly diet. Remember when the Europeans began the slave trade in the 15 century, the diet of newly enslaved tribes was the disregarded meats, yes the meat and food that they didn't eat. And furthermore, remember the European enslavers fed their captive workers as cheaply as possible.

So chicken feet, pig feet, chitlins, and cow tongue, hog mogs were all disregarded by the Europeans. So really if you think about it soul food is really slave food and do we really want to continue to pass this way of eating to our children? Really, I think soul food should be good for your body and soul. Soul food should be steamed veggies, brown rice, fruits and organic protein. No one should be eating the diet of a slave, remember our ancestors didn't want to eat this way they were forced to eat that way in order to survive!

The scripture says our food should be our medicine. Well pig feet is not medicine…lol.. laughing out loud. If we as African Americans continue to eat this S.A.A.D. Standard African American Diet we will continue to have the highest numbers of high blood pressure, breast cancer, diabetes, obesity , and almost every other disease that is out there. We must start to change what soul food is. We must change it to be a healthy way of eating. Soul food should be good for the soul. Just some food for thought…lol

Chapter 3

YOU WILL NOT LOSE YOUR SEXY
IF YOU LOSE WEIGHT

Many black women who I have talked to think if they lose weight, they will also lose their sexy. We have a mixed message going on in our heads. On one hand we think having a big butt and thick thighs are sexy, but on the other hand we feel unattractive with all the extra body weight.

Yes, we turn a man's head with our big butts and thighs, but we are paying dearly for it by being overweight and losing our health. Now don't get me wrong, if your big butt and thick thighs are attached to a healthy weight and BMI, then that's great. But if your BMI is over 25 and you are overweight, that is not sexy—it is unhealthy. Being healthy is the new sexy. Eating a well-balanced, healthy diet is the new sexy.

By the way, BMI is your body mass index. You should know what your BMI is. You can go on many weight loss websites and just plug in your weight and height, and it will calculate your body mass index. If it is over 25, then you're overweight.

We black women have to realize that our beauty is not in our butts and thighs. Being beautiful is achieved by the way we love ourselves and take care of ourselves. We really need to start taking care of ourselves. We need to really start loving ourselves.

Chapter 4

BLACK WOMEN LOSE WEIGHT DIFFERENTLY

There was a study that showed that black women lose weight differently than white women?

Recent health studies have determined that black women loose less weight than white women. The reason for this difference was found to be the failure in black women to adapt to European foods which are common in America as well as their inability to burn more calories than white women. These studies proved that after six months of weight loss programs for black and white women under the same diet plans and exercise, the black women lost an average of 8 pounds less than the white women. It therefore; means that black women require more exercise and fewer calories to shed an equal amount of weight compared to white women on less exercise and more calories.

Did you know that there is a national epidemic of obesity? Did you know that research shows that the African American community has the worst track record? The Center for Disease Control (CDC), says that, 52% of Black women and about 30% of Black men are obese. With records like this our communities around the country will continue to suffer from poor health and untimely deaths. But we can change it by educating ourselves. Yes we must start reading and educating ourselves in order to improve our conditions.

Makeisha Lee is best known as a health columnist and nutritional advisor, she has authored a book titled Why Black People Can't Lose Weight: The Psychology, The Challenge, and The Solution To Overall Wellness. The book addresses common lies and misconceptions about diet schemes, and also uncovers the psychology behind why Blacks fall victim to these. You might want to pick up a copy and read it. It is very informative and could help you when developing your tailor-made weight loss plan.

Now let's get down to business! *It's Easy!*

Chapter 5

REALISTIC WEIGHT LOSS GOALS

ere you are again, having the same old discussion all over again, only this time you're really tired of doing the same thing and expecting different results. Didn't Einstein say something like this: "Insanity is doing the same thing over and over again and expecting different results." Are you insane? If your answer is *no* then stop doing the same thing and expecting different results. Do something different this time, and I don't mean changing to a different diet scam or some crazy, wild exercise plan. Maybe it's time for you to be true to yourself. Maybe it's time for you to develop a plan that's tailor-made for you.

Did you know that most weight loss goals are achievable and easy, especially if they are set according to your standards and not from a fitness training program you came across somewhere. You know your body better than anyone, and therefore you are the best person to design a weight loss program for yourself. But your first priority should be getting healthy and preventing health-related issues. The main focus of your weight loss should be to get healthy, and as a result of that you will lose weight.

If you set standards according to your needs and your own body, then you can succeed in losing weight and keeping it off for a lifetime. Many people want to lose weight fast, and this is a problem. Losing weight too fast can be dangerous to your health. Remember, in order to start any diet or exercise program you should consult first with your physician.

Chapter 6

DESIGN YOUR GOALS TO FIT YOU

This might sound like a cliché, but it is important to set reasonable goals that focus on specific achievements. The more specific you are, the easier it becomes to achieve your goals. Your weight loss goals might require you to adopt certain activities, like eating a balanced diet, getting into a personalized fitness regime, and so on. Each of your activities should include a timetable. In most cases, you need to plan your goals beginning with the short-term goals and ending with the long-term goals.

You need to measure your goals according to your activities and your ideal weight parameters. Therefore, you shouldn't plan your weight loss program to be more weight loss in less time. The time frame goal can be to lose about 1 to 2 pounds each week; this translates to between 12 to 25 pounds in about three months. Now, 12 to 25 pounds might not sound like a lot, but it is! That amount of weight loss can mean a different pants size or dress size. So in order to lose about 12 to 25 pounds in three months, you might need to look at how many calories you are consuming per day. There are plenty of websites that can help you figure out how many calories to consume per day in order to lose 12 to 25 pounds within three months. You can also consult with your doctor, a nutritionist or a dietician. And again, if you can't afford a nutritionist or dietician, check with a doctor and collect as much information as you can. In other words, educate yourself and see your doctor.

Chapter 7

LONG-TERM GOALS

ven though short-term goals are relevant in helping you achieve the long-term goals, it is necessary to keep your main focus on the long-term goals. Technically, the long-term goals will keep you focused, since they can be described as the ultimate weight loss achievements; the short-term goals will help in regulating your routine.

Now, when you start developing your long-term plan make sure it is tailored just for you and your schedule. For example, if you have decided that you want to lose 25 pounds in three months, which could be your long-term plan, make sure that the plan fits comfortably into your life schedule. I liked wearing a pedometer because in my own tailor-made plan I wanted to walk at least 5 miles every day, and in order to walk those 5 miles I needed to take about 10,000 steps per day. So I parked far away from any building I was going to enter, I walked 45 minutes each day during my lunch break, and both of these methods seemed to help a lot. Did you know that 10,000 steps is the equivalent of exercising strenuously for 30 minutes, and that walking about 5 miles per day expends 2,000 to 3,500 calories per week?!

Surprisingly, in most settings the biggest enemy of any weight loss program is the candidate herself—yes, YOU! People have tried for a long time to win weight battles with themselves; some have won them while others fell along the way. In the real sense, you need to overcome your cravings, procrastination and lack of motivation by choosing one of the tried and tested formulas, like finding a workout partner, hiring a fitness trainer, or sticking to your diet and exercise program without falling off the wagon. Ultimately, the weight battle can only be won once you have control over your body. This can be achieved by setting goals to convince yourself that *you can do it! Go for it girl!*

Chapter 8

UNDERSTANDING YOUR BODY COMPOSITION

nderstanding your body composition is important in health mat-ters. By definition, body composition is the body's relative amount of fat to fat-free mass. With the ideal body com-position, you will be able to achieve a greater level of wellness and high-quality living.

Body composition is divided into two types of mass: the fat-free mass and the body fat. The fat- free mass is composed of tissues, muscles, bones and water. On the other hand, the body fat is fat contained in the body. Body fat has many important functions, including protection of the internal organs; it is a good source of energy and plays a key role in regulating hormones relevant to body regulation.

Now, there are significant differences between fat and muscles, even though a pound of each weighs the same. One difference is that muscles are much more compact, while fat tends to take up more space. Just think about this for a minute: a boxer can be 5'6", weigh 200 pounds and look wonderful, and yet another 5'6" person can weigh 200 pounds and look fat and out of shape. This is because one has more muscle and the other has more fat. Muscle is much more compact and takes up a lot less space in your body. Sometimes people who need to lose a lot of weight tend to stay away from weight lifting, but it can be a great way of building your muscles and giving you a sleek, trim look. Keep in mind that the amount of weight you lose by lifting weights is less than you'll get from following a good diet plan.

Basically, the body mass index, or BMI, is one of the methods used by medical specialists to determine a healthy weight. The BMI (body mass index) method uses the weight and height of the individual to determine the body's fat. However, for children and adolescents there are other methods of determining a healthy weight. Additionally, the body mass index is a good indicator of other health-related conditions. For instance, experts say, people with high BMIs are more likely to have high blood pressure, cardiovascular disease, sleep apnea and some forms of cancer. Although BMI is an indicator of certain conditions, genetics and lifestyles can also be used to determine the same.

Chapter 9

WEIGHT LOSS WITH NUTRITION

nce you understand the relevance of nutrition, it's easier to improve your overall health. It's likely that you have tried one or more of the popular and eccentric diets, only to realize that you are either regaining more weight or having an unhealthy weight loss experience. Diets are usually viewed as a short time solution to a lifetime problem. But if you change your eating habits for life by choosing nutritional meals for life, you will win and never have to diet again! We should all want to be healthy, and if we eat healthy, we will be healthy in most cases. You really are what you eat. So, what is nutrition? Wikipedia says: "**Nutrition** is the selection of foods and preparation of foods, and their ingestion to be assimilated by the body. By practicing a healthy diet, many of the known health issues can be avoided. [1] The diet of an organism is what it eats, which is largely determined by the perceived palatability of foods." In other words, again, you are what you eat!

In essence, good nutrition shouldn't be viewed as a part-time hassle that requires occasional participation. It should be approached as a part and parcel of your life. Nutrition is life. If you can maintain a well-balanced diet, you can rest assured that a healthy lifestyle will come naturally. The widely accepted notion that good nutrition is more of a weight loss mechanism should be replaced with a positive attitude towards living a full, healthy and successful life. You can find tons of information on the web about nutrition and nutritional meal plans. In addition, don't forget to ask your doctor if he or she can help you in this area.

Many people view eating healthy as a temporary thing, but it should be something you do on a regular basis. Eating healthy should be a lifestyle. It should be something you do every single day, and eating poorly should be something you do on a temporary basis. I want to emphasize it again: eating poorly should be something we do once in a while, and it should be temporary. If you find yourself eating healthy most of the time, weight loss will be one of the perks, and another perk will be that you will be able to keep the weight off.

Chapter 10

GOOD CARBOHYDRATES VERSUS BAD CARBOHYDRATES

Most people keep asking the question whether carbohydrates (carbs) are bad for you. In essence, some experts say, carbs are only considered bad for you if you eat excessive amounts. Remember the scripture say "every thing in moderation". Let me get back on track, I don't want to go to church on yall…lol.. Laughing out loud! Carbs are divided into simple and complex carbs; health professionals have further described them as bad and good carbs, respectively. The bad carbs are regarded as such because they are fast and easy to digest and they provide short-lived energy. They can be found in candies, cakes, white breads, white rice, white sugars and foods that contain refined sugars. One of my doctors told me to just stay away from anything white…lol.. laughing out loud, he was referring to food. Now, the good carbohydrates (the complex ones) are rich in starches and fibers. They are better than simple carbohydrates because they are more difficult to digest, and that means you stay fuller for a longer time. They are found in legumes, whole grains, fruits and vegetables. Additionally, they are rich in minerals such as zinc, vitamin E and magnesium. For better nutrition, your overall carbohydrate intake should be moderate; also, try to take in more of the complex carbs than the simple carbs.

Now, I know you have heard of low-glycemic carbohydrates, right? Low-glycemic carbs are digested into the body slowly, which means there is a sustained release of sugars in the blood. Furthermore, the low-glycemic foods produce either a minimal spike or no spike at all in circulating blood sugar levels. In addition, eating these carbs means less production of body fat and subsequently lower lipids, which translates to individuals being generally less hungry between meals. If you eat a lot of high-glycemic carbs, it's likely that it will increase your caloric intake from 60 to 70 percent, at least according to reliable studies. People who eat high-glycemic carbs tend to eat at least 200 calories more between meals than those who eat low-glycemic foods.

On the other hand, dieters tend to take in high fiber foods as a means of natural well-being, and of course, as part of their weight loss programs. In most cases, the best high fiber eating plan, in my opinion, will include a lot of natural foods such as whole grains, vegetables, fruits and high fiber cereals. By including a high fiber eating plan in your weight loss program you will be able to reduce your fat intake. You might also want to think about including antioxidant high fiber foods into your program. Studies show that an antioxidant high fiber diet helps to boost our immunity, and also fights off any elements that might damage cells. The antioxidant high fiber choices should include dark green vegetables, grains and fruits. The high fiber diet is great for vegans or vegetarians as well.

Chapter 11

PROTEINS, PROTEINS, PROTEINS

There is so much to say about our protein intake. But what are proteins? Wikipedia says: "**Proteins** are essential nutrients for the human body. [1] They are one of the building blocks of body tissue, and can also serve as a fuel source. As a fuel, proteins contain 4 kcal per gram, just like and unlike lipids, which contain 9 kcal per gram. The most important aspect and defining characteristic of protein from a nutritional standpoint is its amino acid composition. [2]"

So now that we know what proteins are, let's make some sense of it. Proteins tend to burn more calories than other types of energy sources. The source of proteins can come from dairy products, grains, fish or meat, and vegetables. Yes, you can find protein in vegetables, too. Proteins are responsible for the production of stronger bones and muscles, and a stronger immune system. On the other hand, eating too much high-protein food might cause an increase in cholesterol levels and could even put a strain on your kidneys, which could lead to a loss of calcium from the bones. While we know that meats like chicken, turkey, and beef contain protein, many people don't realize that many vegetables also contain protein. Reliable studies show that eating vegetables containing protein will not cause cholesterol levels to increase, or put a strain on your kidneys. Here are some veggies that contain protein:

Peas - Each half-cup contains three and a half grams of protein.

Spinach - You'll find three grams of protein in a half cup of spinach.

Baked potato - Another stealth source of protein? Potatoes! A medium-sized one contains three grams.

Broccoli - Broccoli's not just filled with fiber (2.6 grams per half cup)—it's also a great source of protein, with two grams per serving.

Brussels sprouts - These little green guys get a bad rap, but they're actually nutritional superstars: each half-cup packs two grams of protein, along with 247 milligrams of potassium and 110 micrograms of vitamin K.

Chapter 12

CREATING A EASY MEAL PLAN

reating your own tailor-made meal plan is a personal exercise. This means that you have to create a plan that works around you and your family's schedule, personal tastes, work schedules and workout preferences. The initial step is to choose a budget that fits with your personal food choices. Make sure your custom diet takes into account your weight loss goals. Of course, you will need to research some of the popular diets plans that seem to be working for others like you. There are some pertinent questions that you'll need to ask yourself when you create your diet plan. For instance, you'll need to understand your preferred frequency of eating meals, how much time you spend on meal preparation, what kind of support you will need to get through your weight loss goals and stick to your diet plan, and so on.

For example:
1. Ground beef recipes with less than 300 calories per serving - they are good for a dinner party or for a quick meal.
2. Chili recipes - they are good for heating-up at the last minute and they are full of flavor and nutrition.
3. Casseroles - they can be baked with fillings and you won't have to worry about weight gain as well.

4. Luscious cakes - with only about 250 calories per serving they will surely help you lose weight.
5. Low calorie breakfasts - if you choose these recipes for your breakfasts, you will be able to fill your tummy without adding on much weight.

Make sure you do your research and design a meal plan that fits your life.

Chapter 13

LET'S GET PHYSICAL

There is no doubt that exercise is one of the main ingredients for good health and weight loss. Now, you may ask, *why do I have to exercise?* Well, exercise plays a key role in maintaining a healthy lifestyle. M ore important, when you exercise, you will have control over your weight, which means that you may be able to suppress any diseases and conditions caused by obesity.

Here's why. First, when you engage in physical exercises, you end up burning calories. Second, exercise can avert diseases and health conditions that might be associated with obesity. Third, exercise can increase the level of happiness in an individual. Yes, that's right; studies show that exercise can actually elevate your mood. Energy is an important aspect of how your body functions, because when you exercise, the body's energy levels are boosted to optimum levels. Studies indicate that people who engage in physical exercise sleep better than those who don't. This can be best explained with the example of an overweight person who has a condition such as sleep apnea. Exercise improves life to a degree that it will be recognizable in your rejuvenated self. Last of all, exercise is simply fun once you get the hang of it. Here are some types of exercises for weight loss.

Aerobic exercises

Aerobic exercises consist of a variety of exercises that require your body to use oxygen, thus the term "aerobic". They can involve walking, running, swimming, cycling, dancing and boxing, among others. The choice of exercise you want to do will depend on the kind of resources you have and on your body weight. For instance, it might be difficult for some overweight people to start a running program because of their body weight. However, they might warm up to such exercises by walking for a period of time, then improving on that by doing more as they continue with their program. Here's some good news - it's nice to know that it doesn't matter if you walk or run, you still end up burning almost the same amount of calories. Swimming and cycling are also fun, especially if you want to develop muscles.

Exercise balls

Some might regard exercise balls as a fad that will fade away as time goes by, as far as workouts are concerned. But for any exercise enthusiast, exercise balls play a significant role in strengthening the torso, and with fewer injuries. Exercise balls are a favorite with most trainers because of their ease of use and for other benefits associated with them. For example, they can be used for increasing your stability and for strengthening the back and abs. They can be used as a bench in weight training, playing or sitting around, abdominal training, flexibility training or during yoga classes.

Lifting weights

There is no better method of strength training than through weight lifting. Understandably, most people who want to lose weight tend to concentrate on cardio exercises more than they do on strength training; that's a good thing, because cardio is necessary for burning fat and developing a lean physique. But I want to emphasize weight lifting because of the benefits associated with it, such as having a faster metabolism, which comes from having more muscle. Muscles are essential for burning a lot of calories. For women, weight lifting will help strengthen our bones, too.

You will see an increase in your endurance, and your overall strength will be built-up as well. Additionally, it will help you improve your coordination and balance. Ultimately it will play a key role in boosting your self-esteem and confidence.

The basics of lifting weight include lifting more weight than you are used to, increasing the weight as you go along, remaining focused on your goals and weight loss targets, and allowing some days for resting and recovery.

Running/jogging outdoors

One of the differences between running and jogging is the intensity. Running is more intense than jogging, and it requires you to burn more kilojoules. Ok, you are probably thinking, what are kilojoules? Here's what the The Heart Foundation says: "The difference between calories and kilojoules is rather like the difference between miles and kilometers. Kilojoules are the metric equivalent of calories; 1 kJ equals 0.2 calories."

Both running and jogging are aerobic exercises as well. You might want to include these types of exercises in your weight loss program. It is necessary to have a medical checkup to determine whether you are fit for these types of exercises, especially if you are older than 40. Other hindrances you might run into can include having a chronic illness, or if you haven't exercised for a long time. Your running should be preceded by brisk walking in the initial days for about 30-minute sessions, for six weeks. You need to warm-up each time you plan on running. The best place to jog or run is in a park or away from major roads and highways. Remember to purchase the proper running shoes and again see your doctor before starting any exercise programs!

Treadmill workouts

One of the common mistakes people make while working out is stepping, jogging or running at a constant speed for twenty to thirty minutes. The other mistake is starting out without pacing or warming up. If the exercises on a treadmill are not properly done, they could lead to injuries or even frustration. In order to exercise safely on a treadmill, you need to always warm-up, increase your workout sessions progressively, and give yourself enough time to cool down; you do not want to hop off a treadmill and then sit down abruptly because it could cause muscle cramps. The exercises should be done in progressive speeds for improvement in your cardiovascular workout, plus you get to work out various muscles as your stride changes.

Cycling

Cycling to lose weight can be described as fun, social, and quite challenging. Anyone can take up cycling since it is a cheap method of working out. It is great for burning calories while it improves your health. It is a wonderful way to achieve your weight goals and fitness. Cycling targets a number of muscle groups, especially in the legs, such as the hamstrings, quadriceps, calves and glutei. Unlike most exercises, pedal power shifts weight from the upper body to the lower body, and as such it offers a great alternative while putting less pressure on the joints. When it comes to cycling, you do not need any special training; after all, most of us can ride a bike comfortably. In a half hour session you can lose between 76 and 670 extra calories. And again I can't stress this enough it is important to see your doctor before starting any kind of exercise programs.

Chapter 14

HOLISTIC WELLNESS AND WEIGHT LOSS

his is one of my favorite subjects. Why? Because holistic medicine is the type of treatment that focuses on the person's entire being, and not specifically on the treatment of symptoms. Like holistic medicine, the holistic approach for weight loss follows a similar path in finding the underlying causes of the problems associated with weight gain. In essence, such procedures can help in achieving a sustainable weight loss program aimed for long-term goals. Even if other weight loss programs fail, you can depend on the holistic methods of weight loss.

The holistic methods will help you understand the causes of your weight woes, while at the same time creating an enlightening path to total weight freedom. First off, it's necessary to state that a weight problem is not actually a disease. However, it can lead to a number of conditions and diseases if it is not properly managed. There are a number of holistic approaches that an individual can follow in a weight loss program, such as positive messages, meditation, visualization, psychotherapy, drinking more water and correct breathing. Let's explore a few of them.

Meditation
There is a certain conviction associated with meditating as a form of treatment. When people meditate, they are able to connect with an

inner spirit and a deep thoughtfulness that lies within them. If they are able to control that element of their sub-consciousness, they are able to free themselves of any hindrances that affect their physical condition. For example, a binge eater can become aware of the cause of her eating problems through a self-realization moment. If the meditation is progressive, she can also take note of significant moments, like when she is hungry or not. The most important thing about meditation is that an individual can tackle the underlying factors which affect her physical issues.

Drinking more water

Drinking more water falls into the holistic category because it uses less familiar, conventional tactics than just changing your diet or exercising. For one, drinking more water during the initial days of weight loss is useful in replenishing the body's water content that is lost due to dehydration. The process of dehydration slows down the process of burning calories, and as such, you need to drink a lot of water. There are toxins produced during weight loss, especially from burning calories. Therefore, you need a lot of water to flush out some of these toxins in the body. Dehydration also causes a reduction in blood volume, which translates to less oxygen in the blood.

A high fiber diet is strongly recommended for the maintenance of a healthy diet; however, this type of food can lead to constipation if your body lacks vital fluids such as water. Water is necessary for the maintenance of muscle tone and for helping muscle contractions. In addition, water helps to lubricate your joints.

Breathing

Oxygen is a crucial component in metabolism and thus in the exercises you do. In essence, the more oxygen you have in your blood stream, the faster your metabolism will be. Obviously, oxygen is obtained in the body through breathing. Surprisingly though, people have not mastered the art of breathing while they exercise. In reality, people tend to take either shallow breaths or to hold their breath in intense situations. As you can see, an individual who is in a weight loss program needs to learn how to breathe correctly in order to have more benefical exercises. In essence, you might not lose weight through the breathing process itself, but correct breathing will facilitate the weight loss process. You can learn how to breathe fresh air by standing, sitting down or lying down in nature. You would require the help of an expert to make sure that you do these breathing exercises properly.

Now take a deep breath and say, *I can do this. I am going to get healthy. I love myself.*

Author's final thoughts

So now you have some information that may help you get healthy and lose weight, too. You can even develop your own tailor-made plan of action. You don't need to follow someone else's plan because it might not work for you long-term. Weight loss is a way to regain your health.

Loving yourself is all about being healthy as you possibly can. Loving yourself is about first of all putting yourself first. Yes you have to put yourself first before you can help anyone else. If you get healthy, your children will be healthy, your husband will be healthy. Getting healthy is contagious! Contagious in a good way.

Make sure you do your homework and check out different websites, read as much as you can and make sure you consult with your doctor.

As for me, ten years after breast cancer, I am healthier than I have been in a long time. I am still a size 6, and I love it! And I still got my sexy… LOL. Laughing out loud! Peace.

Here are some of my secrets to weight loss.
1. Don't eat after 7:00 pm. You may ask why? Well if you eat your last meal before 7:00pm you are giving your body ample time to digest the food.
2. Drink a glass of water with lemon every morning before a meal this will I think it helps your body to digest anything that might be left over and I have read its good for the liver.

3. Find yourself a good multivitamin. It will help with the nourishment your body needs.
4. Drink plenty of water to stay hydrated.
5. Exercise at least 30 minutes a day even if it's a 15 minute walk twice a day.